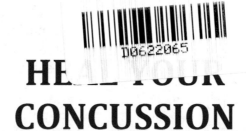

HEAL YOUR
CONCUSSION

21 Days to Brain Health

Dr. Joanny Liu, TCMD, RAc, PEng

ISBN: 978-0-9940150-2-0

Medical Disclaimer

The information presented in this book is the result of years of study, research, practical experience and clinical research by the author. The information in this book, by necessity, is of general nature and not a substitute for an evaluation or treatment by a competent medical practitioner of Chinese Medicine and Chinese Psychology. If you believe you are in need of medical intervention please see a certified Dr of Acupuncture or Dr of Traditional Chinese Medicine or Dr of Oriental Medicine.

Cover graphic attribution: Image by A Health Blog on Flickr, used under the Creative Commons license.The image was flipped to face outward to the right.Thank you!

FREE Audiobook!

If you would like to listen to the audiobook version of *Heal Your Concussion* while you follow along with this ebook, you can download it for free for a limited time by clicking on this link:

www.drjoanny.com/free-audiobook-offer-hyc

Table of Contents

Introduction
"I Got A Concussion!"

The last thing I ever expected was to pick up a call from my son, Nolan, 29, and hear his story of woe.

He said, "Mom, I was hit so hard in the head, I went *BLIND!*"

Then he told me what happened.

He was playing soccer and he was marking his man on his side of the field, when unbeknownst to him, a teammate kicked the ball towards him. He was so focused on the opposition that he had NO idea that the ball was coming towards him. He was completely caught off guard and was smucked hard on the right side of his head. He dropped to the ground!

His teammates got him off to the sidelines, where he sat sorting things out. That's when he realized he couldn't see. Imagine what might've been going through his mind. The fear. Maybe panic. The disorientation. SUDDENLY, everything changed.

He doesn't know how long he sat there. Maybe it was 10 minutes, maybe 20. But when his eyesight finally came back he went back on the field! Even though he wasn't feeling well.

His team was short handed that day. He felt responsible. He felt like a pylon but at least some of his teammates could have a short break.

After the game, he drove home. When he got home, the headaches started. He decided he would stop doing ALL extracurricular activities. The only thing he couldn't stop doing was work – he's a busy professional engineer with responsibilities.

He tried to deal with his concussion by himself, after all he's a grown man.

By the time he called me, it was more than 2 weeks since his concussion. His symptoms only got worse. He wasn't sleeping. He wasn't eating. He had headaches almost all the time, ranging from dull to stabbing pain. He was miserable and definitely suffering.

He finally asked me for help.

I told him in no uncertain terms, "Ok, then you have to do everything I tell you to do."

This was in late August. We worked with each other for a few weeks and he improved right from the beginning. Within a few short weeks he was back at light practices. He kept improving and then he did what he usually does all winter – he plays indoor soccer, skis in the Canadian Rockies and plays in a pool league.

Nolan has had NO relapses. NO headaches. NO eye problems. At the time of this writing, he's been Concussion Free for about 28 months.

Make no mistake. You CANNOT afford to be passive about your brain injury. You CAN recover from one. I'm going to outline some of the most important things we did together to make my son STRONG again.

You have the key to Brain Health right in front of you NOW.

I know that life changed the minute you experienced your concussion. Maybe you've had to quit your job. Maybe you've had to give up ALL the things you love to do. You've reduced your expectations. You're functioning at a much lower level than you ever imagined. I know it's TOUGH and downright disheartening that a once talented resourceful and creative person like you could be so sidelined by life.

BUT, that's why you MUST start thinking outside-of-the-box, because the truth is:

Your concussion is temporary.

You have to use your brain to heal your brain! This is what neuroplasticity or brain plasticity is – changing your brain. You can do it consciously - or unconsciously, which right now is keeping you in the same place.

The value of working through the Ten Steps is to prove to yourself just how capable and dynamic a human being you REALLY are!

You are a problem solver. You will free your mind of doubt. Your mind will let go of what you thought was IMPOSSIBLE. And that includes recovering successfully from your concussion.

You will grow confident, because you will feel safe. And then you will heal FASTER than ever. Healing occurs in the mind first. Your work in these following chapters will show you how to enter FLOW. Flow is constant focus. It suspends time. It suspends disbelief. This is where you feel the most alive and the most accomplished.

Flow is where you go when you want to heal when you become determined *and relaxed.*

Choose deliberately and you will heal your concussion by yourself. With just a little of my help. Just like my son did.

Every day, you can make a different choice. If you choose today, you can recover from a concussion as fast as YOU WANT. You can recover from post-concussive syndrome because it's never too late if you know HOW and WHY.

Don't let yourself off the hook. Don't abandon yourself. You can instead heal your concussion. Just follow the Ten Steps I have for you.

And one more thing! CELEBRATE every single milestone you hit in these Ten Steps. CELEBRATE every victory! No matter how big or small. You will make progress, so celebrate each Step you complete, every goal you reach, every time you feel good again, be aware of it as a victory and CELEBRATE!

CHAPTER 1
The 3 Giant Myths About Concussions

Here are the Three Giant Myths about concussions that actually prolong your suffering.

1. You have to get an X-ray.

2. You can't do anything except rest and wait it out.

3. You can't speed up the healing process.

Myth No. 1: Get an X-Ray

In fact, an X-ray only shows bone. A fractured skull hardly ever occurs with a concussion, but a concussion can happen with a fractured skull. It takes an awful lot of force to break bone, so most likely you don't have a fractured skull. A concussion is mostly about some impairment in functionality, not brain structure. Currently MRIs and other scanning machines can't reliably detect any visible problems with the soft tissue of the brain. It's a waste of time and money.

Instead it's better to look at these signs of concussions. Mind you, you should be getting more than one of these symptoms to be sure that you've got one.

- Headaches.

- Nausea.

- Vomiting or the urge to vomit.

- Insomnia.

- Emotional upset or being more sensitive.

- Mental confusion or lack of mental clarity.

- Vision problems.

These are the most common symptoms of a concussion. This is what you should look for.

Myth No. 2: Complete Rest

Rest. This is yesterday's "treatment." Stay at home from school and work. Stay in a dark room and do nothing. If you fall asleep, wake up. Which kind of contradicts the first piece of advice. In any case, none of these things are "treatments" but it is about waiting for chance to heal.

By doing nothing you could actually suffer even longer or even if you recover you could have a relapse. One mother told me that she just simply could not see her active 11-year-old son staying put in a dark room doing nothing for days on end. Another told me that her daughter was still suffering from post-concussive symptoms a year after the original concussion.

They were looking for a better way. There is a BETTER WAY.

Myth No. 3: You Can't Speed Up the Healing Process

If you don't know what to do about a concussion in the first place then you certainly won't know how to speed up the healing process. So in these pages I'm going to show you what to do. You won't need any expensive machinery or drugs or intervention to heal. You will just need your mind, a pencil and paper or your computer. And of course your time and undivided attention for the next 21 days as you work through the assignments I have for you.

Here are your ingredients for success:

1. Desire. Is your desire GREATER than any fear you or someone else feels about going through the healing process you're about to take? Yes or No.

2. Determination. Will you give the healing process the time and resources to work on it? Yes or No.

3. Persistence. Will you stick to the healing process to recover completely? Yes or No.

4. Trust. Will you keep going even if it looks difficult? Yes or No.

Chances are you said "Yes!" to each question. Your brain has already started to heal. Revisit these questions when you get discouraged. These are your four ingredients that will ensure your success: Leave your concussion behind in the past where it belongs!

CHAPTER 2
What We Know About The Brain TODAY

It's really important that you understand that you can use your brain to heal the brain. If you had a broken arm, would you allow it to atrophy? Of course not. You'd be going to therapy to exercise it. You'd use it again. So the best way to heal a traumatic brain injury is to use the brain.

The truth is this: Healing your concussion isn't difficult. The reason why there's so much fear in the news and in the medical establishment is that they don't know how to help you. You can take the steps I outline here in this book for you. Apply yourself. Follow through with the NEW life skills I'm going to teach you in this little book.

Brain Science or neuroscience has changed a lot in the last 25 years.

Scientists used to think that you couldn't improve your brain in any way, that the brain you had you're stuck with for the rest of the your life. They used to think that if you lost brain cells, you couldn't get more.

Through the miracle of functional brain scans, like functional MRIs, of living brains, we can see what happens in the brain. We can attach electrodes on your head and ask you questions and see which parts of the brain are working. We can see how you create a state of mind within your living brain.

Today, we know that

1. The brain is very plastic. We can change it. This is exciting because this means YOU have BIG possibilities!

2. The brain can be repaired. It can grow NEW and MORE brain cells.

Brain cells are also called neurons. At first they could be standalone, but they can't act alone. Neurons must be connected and when they are, they act in a coordinated manner in groups called Neural Networks.

Neural networks develop as a result of continuous activation between neurons. They stick around because of *strong emotional connection and repetition*. This is how memories are created. This is how you memorize something. Memories are hard wired neural networks in your brain because they are activated many, many times.

Emotion is very important in the process of memorization. If you can't find an emotional reason to remember something, you won't remember it. Emotion is the juice that makes memories stick. If you stop using a memory, after awhile those networks will be "pruned" away. That's why you forget. If it's unimportant, if there's no emotion connected to it and you don't bring it up often, your brain won't store it.

Let's look at an analogy. We have two neurons. In the beginning, they're neighbors that don't know each other. Neuron A needs a tool from his neighbor and goes over to introduce himself. He asks if he can borrow the tool. The connection is made with Neuron B. Neuron B obliges and hands over the tool. Later Neuron A comes back with the borrowed tool and is very grateful and happy. They strike up a friendship and they start doing things together. Now they have a little neural network between the two of them.

They start inviting other neighbors next door to them and they start a tool-lending co-op. They keep making connections with more neighbors. They get to know each other better and better and pretty soon they have a growing network. Each time they meet someone new, they benefit. The more they talk to each neighbor, the stronger the connection gets. Then they have a reliable network of neurons that they can get help from. Every one is happy.

Now let's talk about two people who aren't getting along. What if one of the neighbors was late getting the tool back to the lender. What if neighbor A decided he was going to keep the tool and not return it? Neighbor B, the lender, might grow distrustful. He might think that every one is like this. The price he pays as he thinks about it is stress and upset. If he continues to feel and think repeatedly over and over, he creates a negative neural network.

Thought. Emotion. Repetition. Memory.

CHAPTER 3
You Are an Emotional Being Because Your Brain Is an Emotional Organ

In the previous chapter, the lender got all upset and stressed out from his experience. Stress is prolonged negative feelings that are compounded by negative thoughts. If you're upset over something over time, then you're firing the same neural networks over and over.

You're human and you're an emotional being. So you feel the emotions that are attached to a given situation. You can't help it. This is your nature. Here is the role of your emotions: They tell you whether you like or dislike something that's happening right now.

They are meant to be released quickly. So a short stint where you might have a strong negative reaction to something won't harm your body or your brain. If you can do something positive and constructive right away then you'll calm down quickly.

But for many people, feeling unhappy becomes a long term HABIT. They tend to let these bad stressful feelings fester and grow. This is what creates problems. The more you focus on those unsettling circumstances, the more upset you get, just like neighbor B did.

Stress HARMS the brain!

Stress is prolonged negative feelings that are compounded by negative thoughts and feelings. Those thoughts and feelings trigger the Sympathetic Nervous System, which releases the stress hormones, cortisol and adrenaline. These stress hormones flood both your body and the brain.

This is what stress does to the brain:

The hippocampus is the part of the brain that deals with memories, learning and emotions. *It's also where most new brain cells are created because you're creating memories.*

A healthy hippocampus tells another part of the brain, the hypothalamus, to stop releasing cortisol when it reaches a certain level. This is why you calm down relatively quickly when you're upset. Normally, you'll recover quickly.

But when you're often unhappy (stressed out or upset), your body is going to secrete stress hormones constantly. Too many stress hormones damage the hippocampus cells to the point that they can't tell the hypothalamus to stop secreting cortisol, *so more stress hormones are released which causes a vicious cycle.*

If you keep thinking and feeling bad about your concussion, you're creating more of the same neurons. *As you keep reliving your injury over and over, you're building connections in your brain between individual brain cells and groups of brain cells.* If you're only focused on what's bad in your life then you're also NOT creating new neurons. The existing ones become networked – so you're building neural networks and hardwiring the negative things. You reinforce them by thinking the same thoughts and having the same feelings over and over. *And your brain starts craving them!* This is how you form habits (good and bad).

BUT here's the GOOD News!

Positive thoughts and feelings also feed off each other. Your brain is favorably affected by positive thoughts and feelings. In this case, hormones such as oxytocin, from the Parasympathetic Nervous System are secreted. Oxytocin has a calming effect.

You can reverse the harm done anytime you want. And that's where this book comes in. You will learn how to deal with your life, your brain and your body. You will feel SOOTHED and CONFIDENT and in CONTROL again.

"We have to stop our most natural way of thinking and feeling (and feeling and thinking) to repattern the brain." ~ Dr. Joe Dispenza, *Evolve Your Brain*

Throughout the day, you're not really thinking because you're automatically acting on programmed neural networks that are already hardwired in your brain. It only takes one thought or something that reminds you of something to activate a programmed set of responses and behaviors. It feels natural and normal. Even if it makes you feel bad.

I remind you: *your concussion is temporary.*

The key is to learn how to calm down and turn on the right kind of Brain Plasticity. You want fresh new cells that come from positive constructive experiences that will heal. This is what my regimen, Activated Constructive Thinking™ is all about. You will be LEARNING new things. You will be ADAPT-ING and CHANGING your brain in a very structured and per-sonalized way. This is the KEY to healing your concussion.

This is the greatest connection you'll ever make: *Your psy-chology and your physiology are intimately intertwined and cannot be separated.* When you work on each of the Ten Steps that I have for you, you're going to be changing your mind. This is what Activated Constructive Thinking™ will do for you. You will think differently. You will form positive habits. You will be rewiring your brain. The result is: You will feel confident. You will feel safe.

The secret to your success is a happy life with new happy mem-

ories.

You're going to learn my secrets to become happy with purpose. In order for something to change, then there must be creativity applied to a problem to solve it. *Your concussion is just another problem that you can solve.*

CHAPTER 4
Rate Your Concussion

First, you must establish a benchmark for yourself. You must know where you are now before you step up into the program. The reason for this is very simple: You have to compare how you feel later on to how you feel right now before you begin the work in earnest. That's how you'll know if you're making progress.

On a scale of 0 to 10, I want you to rate the progress achieved during the healing process. It will boil down to your symptoms disappearing and how long they stay away. We're not into half measures here. Progress is made when you work the system, Activated Constructive Thinking™, in this book. Follow it and you'll get results!

Here's what the basic scale looks like:

0   1   2   3   4   5   6   7   8   9   10   N/A

Of course, the ratings you choose are purely subjective. And for some of these categories, they may not apply to your situation, so choose N/A if that is the case. Or if you find none of these descriptions exactly describes your condition, then you pick a number and write down the meaning of it to you, thus personalizing.

After filling these out, get to work ASAP and monitor yourself after every step. Be patient. Keep working. Aren't you worth it? Begin NOW.

Rate the frequency of your headaches.

0   1   2   3   4   5   6   7   8   9   10   N/A

0 means no headaches. (This is your goal.)

1 means 1 headache per day, which starts and stops. So we're talking about separate headaches

2 means 2 headaches per day, which start and stop and then start up again.

8 – 9 mean there are too many to count OR you have one continuous headache that is omnipresent but mild.

10 means either too many to count OR you can't stand having headaches, which makes you want to jump off a cliff!

Rate the severity of pain in your headaches.

0   1   2   3   4   5   6   7   8   9   10   N/A

0 means no pain. (This is your goal.)

1 means you can barely feel it.

10 means you want to jump off a cliff!

Rate the severity of the feeling of nausea.

0   1   2   3   4   5   6   7   8   9   10   N/A

0 means no nausea. (This is your goal.)

1 means you can barely feel it.

10 means you want to jump off a cliff!

Rate the severity of vomiting (or desire to vomit if it doesn't happen).

0   1   2   3   4   5   6   7   8   9   10   N/A

0 means no vomiting or no urge to vomit. (This is your goal.)

1 means you barely want to.

10 means you want to jump off a cliff!

Rate the severity of insomnia.

0   1   2   3   4   5   6   7   8   9   10   N/A

0 means no insomnia; you're sleeping well. (This is your goal.)

1 means you experience sleeplessness at night once a week.

10 means you're not getting any sleep at all!

Rate the improvement to mental clarity.

0   1   2   3   4   5   6   7   8   9   10   N/A

0 means no clarity; you feel confused all the time.

8 – 9 means you're extremely aware of what has made you sick or injured in the past. (This is your goal.)

10 means you feel in control of your life because you understand the true cause of disease.

Rate the severity of vision problems.

0   1   2   3   4   5   6   7   8   9   10   N/A

0 means no problems with eyes or vision. (This is your goal.)

1 means you experience problems rarely with your eyes.

2 and beyond means you're experiencing more frequent problems with vision.

10 means you're continually experiencing problems with your eyes and vision.

NOTE: After you've created this first rating, put it away. Its purpose is to show you where you are today. But I don't want you looking at it every day. This is your "old" self and is no longer relevant. You will only bring it out on the last day when you finish this Activated Constructive Thinking™ Program and compare it to the most recent one you do.

Rate yourself after you've completed each exercise in this book or at the end of one or two days. Put those away. Celebrate any victories! Keep moving.

From this point onwards you will focus on what you are becoming – a brain-healthy person. That is the most important thing you can do for yourself.

Now, let's begin!

CHAPTER 5
Step 1: Pay Attention to Your Self-Talk

Day 1.

Did you rate your concussion yet? If not, do it now before going further.

Negative self-talk is sabotage. You believe that you have no control over your life. You make yourself believe this lie. No matter where it originated, it doesn't matter. It's time to take negative self-talk out of your life for good.

You DO have control, you know. You have control over your body, your mind, your life. So I want you to start thinking, "I am in control of healing my concussion." Whenever you find yourself telling yourself lies, such as, "I can't do this", but you want to be well, repeat the sentence. Every time you hear you're no good or it won't work, repeat the sentence.

"I am in control of healing my concussion."

You're going to change your brain by changing your thoughts and emotions. Remember what happens in the brain when you're stressed out (feeling intensely unhappy, afraid)? It gets flooded with stress hormones from the Sympathetic Nervous System. You're going to learn how to turn on the Parasympathetic Nervous System. This will trigger the calming hormone, oxytocin. This is what you want - calm.

But in order to have LASTING effects, you must solve your problems and I know you are hot and bothered.

So every day you will work on yourself using the Ten Steps. You will be required to review each step each day as you progress because you WILL make progress.

Being a tire kicker of your life is like being a guy at a bus stop who hasn't bothered to look up the transit schedule. In this day and age of the internet, there is no reason not to know when to expect the next bus to come along. What if you have to wait an hour in between buses during non-rush hours? You could've missed the bus within minutes but you didn't even know that. Now you're at the bus stop not knowing when the next one comes.

Is that your life right now? Waiting and not knowing?

Here's your chance to take control.

The following chapters are your steps to Concussion Freedom. Spend one day, up to three days, with the concepts of each chapter. Understand the IMPORTANCE of each instruction. And make it your own.

You can feel much better in 21 days. It is possible for you to be free of your concussion in 21 days. You are proceeding with the secret sauce. Take control of your mind, your emotions, your brain, your stress levels and your happiness levels.

Start saying to yourself, several times a day, "I am in control of healing my concussion", every hour for 5 minutes or in a cluster when you remember. Immerse yourself in a feeling that is happy or full of relief – whatever positive feeling you can muster very time you repeat, "I am in control of healing my concussion." Say it like you mean it (SILYMI)!

Keep up the good work!

Begin NOW.

CHAPTER 6
Step 2: How To Heal with Food

Day 2

1. Remind yourself a few times a day, "I am in control of healing my concussion." Repeat every hour for 5 minutes or every time you remember all day long. Say it like you mean it (SILYMI)

Keep up the good work!

When you've completed this step, use the rate form from Chapter 4 to rate how you feel.

Food is much more than just vitamins, minerals, proteins, fats and carbohydrates. Foods have an EFFECT on you. The Chinese discovered these effects thousands of years ago. We still use this information along with the principles of Chinese Medicine and Chinese Psychology. So this is another skill you're going to learn.

Remember, LEARNING and PRACTICING new things over and over will change your brain. You will create new neural networks and you will fire them over and over, but only IF you practice over and over.

Food is your medicine. Here's how to do it in a snap shot.

You need to eat differently to:

- Clear your mind

- Keep Warm From the Inside Out

- Speed up healing and know which foods slow down healing

First, I want to tell you a story. I live in Calgary, Alberta and we have a very famous annual festival every July, called The Calgary Stampede, which has been dubbed "The Greatest Outdoor Show on Earth!" Sometimes, one of the local newspapers sends an intrepid reporter to the Stampede Exhibit Grounds, so that he eats and almost lives there for the entire 10-day festival. Of course there's LOTS of junk food there.

Before he headed out to the grounds, a medical team examined and recorded all of his "vital" signs. That's the benchmark. Then he went out and ate all day long at the Stampede. He was required to come in for regular checkups. As time past, they found that some of his vitals, like his blood pressure, had gotten worse. He also felt grumpy and more irritable than normal. His weight stayed the same because he walked the grounds all day long, but he didn't feel like himself.

The lesson: What you eat affects how you feel. Keep that in mind. Definitely one of the things that a concussion does to you, is you feel muddled. Your thinking isn't as sharp. You may feel lethargic, confused. Don't make it worse. Make it better.

So definitely cut out junk food - you should anyways!

Also cut out alcohol for the time being. Alcohol also muddles the mind. So you might as well abstain until you've healed.

Now look at food differently.

Keep warm from the inside out. Certain foods are cooling, such as RAW vegetables, RAW fruits, shellfish and of course anything that you take out of the refrigerator or freezer. For foods kept in cold storage it's obvious. But the Chinese observed how foods AFFECT people. So they defined foods energetically cold BECAUSE they made people FEEL cold.

For instance, tea is cooling. Even when you drink hot tea, after a while you will feel cooler. That's why people in southeast Asia drink hot tea in their hot climate. Hot tea makes them sweat! It's cooling the body.

Other foods have an EFFECT of heat on the body. These are warming foods. For instance, how do you feel after eating a piece of ginger? But cold foods can be made to have a WARMING EFFECT on the body if they're cooked. So, having said that vegetables are cold or cooling, they should be cooked. Vegetables contain the lion's share of natural vitamins and minerals for your body. Eat them cooked for maximum nutrient absorption too.

To make it simple for you, here are simple guidelines for you for the specific case of concussions.

Please do these:

Eat all your food *cooked* until you've completely healed.

Limit the amount of fruit you eat to just one or two servings everyday until you're healed, either lightly cooked or store fruit at room temperature. For example, a small red apple is a serving.

Limit the amount of sour foods you eat. Most fruit is sweet *and* sour. Other sour foods are vinegar and ketchup.

Eat *LOTS of hearty soups and stews* for added warmth and easy digestion.

Drink all beverages either room temperature, warm or hot.

Please cut these out:

Stop eating junk food.

Stop consuming alcoholic beverages until you've completely healed.

Stop eating foods that have a COLD effect on your body, such as salads, raw vegetables and fruits, ice cream, sushi and sashimi until you've completely healed.

Stop drinking *ice cold drinks* such as water, fruit juice, soft drinks and milk for the time being. (Cut out soft drinks: bad for you!)

If you'd like more information, my other books, *Knock OUT Concussions* and *Rapid Injury Recovery: How Elite Athletes Use Sports Psychology to Heal FAST and Have a Long Stable Career*, have much more in depth approach and explanation to this and many topics. You're welcome to explore these books too.

Now, get your food cupboards in order! Take the first steps with your next meal.

CHAPTER 7
Step 3: What are your priorities?

Day 3

- "I am in control of healing my concussion." (SILYMI)

- Get used to eating Food that is your Medicine.

All day long. Keep up the good work!

When you've completed this step, use the rate form from Chapter 4 to rate how you feel.

A priority is something that is regarded as more important than another. I want you to pay attention to the things in your life that are important to you. List them on a sheet of paper or in a spreadsheet on your computer or mobile device.

After you've listed them, I want you to read them over and number them. Let's say you wrote down 10 things. Choose the most important thing and put 10 next to it, so that it has the highest priority. Then go on through the list and place a number between 1 and 10 next to it. Some items on your list will have the same priority.

When you've done that, choose the top 5. These are your highest priorities.

Now, I want you to examine each one and ask these questions:

Is this priority related to my health? Yes or No.

Is this priority related to my family? Yes or No.

Is this priority related to my career/job? Yes or No.

After examining them, what do you see?

If none of them are related to your health, you have discovered a problem. You have decided consciously or unconsciously that you DON'T matter.

Correct this oversight now. In order to become well again, you must CHOOSE your health as *your number one priority right now*. Even if it is in the top five, as long as it is not your NUMBER ONE top priority you have to make it that way. By thinking this way, your brain will be focused on a solution. Get everything on your side, especially your brain. This is another way to help your brain heal itself.

For the rest of your life, your priorities should look like this:

Your Number ONE priority is Your Health.

Your Number TWO priority is Your Family.

Your Number THREE priority is Your Career/Job.

Why is Your Health so important? Because if you take care of Number ONE, then you will be around to take care of number two and three. That's why! If you're too sick to work, can you take care of yourself? If you have a family, can you do a good job taking care of them? NO. That's why you have to take care of yourself first. Be healthy for you and you'll be there for your family, your fiends and your colleagues at work.

Don't underestimate the importance of this part. It's extremely critical that there is a change in priorities and therefore, attitude. It is said that many people, at the end of their lives, regret not having spent more time with their families. Many people may have died rich, but they were alone. They sacrificed everything outside of their work for their wealth because they didn't understand that the people around them would never understand why they worked so hard.

Set your priorities straight from now on.

I want you to think deeply about you being Number ONE. Remind yourself every hour for 5 minutes in silence or say aloud: "My health is my top Number One priority." You are declaring that you are indeed worth it! That's a BIG reason to celebrate! Begin NOW.

CHAPTER 8
Step 4: What Do You Really Want?

Day 4:

Remember these:

- "I am in control of healing my concussion." (SILYMI)
- Keep eating Food that is your Medicine.
- "My health is my top Number One priority." (SILYMI)

All day long. Keep it going – you got it in you!

When you've completed this step, use the rate form from Chapter 4 to rate how you feel.

A want is a desire for something. What is it that you desire the most? What do you want to do AFTER you're finally free of your concussion that you can't do now? Write them down. To go after those things that you want, you must set goals. A goal is the object of your ambition or effort. It's an aim or a desired result.

Without a goal you are like a ship without a rudder. You go wherever the current takes you. You are letting others and circumstances dictate your life. Not good, is it? You want more control right? So the first step to taking back control of your brain and the rest of your life is to set goals.

A goal gives you direction. It gives you purpose.

Answer these questions first. Please answer them honestly.

Do you feel you deserve to live a good healthy life? Yes or No.

Do you want to recover from concussions faster, with certainty? Yes or No.

Do you want to discover how you can prevent concussions? Yes or No.

Do you want to live your life on your own terms? Yes or No.

Chances are excellent that you answered, "Yes" to these questions. If you did, it means that you have a clear idea about what you want. Clarity is what you're after.

Now let's get down to specifics.

When you create your goals:

1. Be sure they're YOUR goals, not someone else's. I'm sure you'll agree that when you chose your own goals, you were much more successful at achieving them. This shouldn't be a surprise. *When it's what you want, you feel good about it and you WANT to have it.* Don't let someone else dictate to you! Be sure to ignore someone else's input.

2. Here's an idea to help you brainstorm: What do you spend time complaining about? What do you spend time blaming others for?

3. Write down your goals to make them more real to you. Writing them down shows commitment and also integrity. Writing them down shows your BRAIN what you want it to do.

4. Look at each goal that you've written down. How does the first one make you feel? Happy? Inspired? Excited? Good. Keep those. Or dread? Or neutral, nothing at all? Ok, throw those out. If you feel bad or nothing, then these aren't the right goals for you. Take them off the list.

5. Finally, get it down to 2 or 3 goals.

6. Look at your goals every morning. This forms an anchor for your brain to focus on. Goals enable you to drive your energy and effort. You're actually telling your conscious and subconscious mind to look for the things that will help you to reach your goals.

It may be that you don't know what you want. It could be that no one has ever asked you what YOU want. Maybe people have always told you what you want, whether you thought so or not. Emotionally that's not a good thing for you because you've allowed others to live their lives through you. You've lost autonomy and self-esteem because you're not thinking for yourself.

If you don't know what you want, then ask yourself, "What do I really want?" Then your brain will be focused on that. Eventually you will start getting ideas. Write them down and sort them out the way I asked you.

This is VERY important.

My son was motivated by three reasons. He wanted to play indoor (fall/winter) soccer which was just a couple of months away. He wanted to ski all winter long and had actually already planned and PAID for six different ski trips. It wasn't just the money he'd lose, but watching his friends go without him that bothered him. He also had to keep working. As a single guy who owns his own home, continuing to be independent and making money was very important to him. My son chose to become healthy again.

Spend up to 2 days working on your goals. You should have a plan for each one and a deadline. Deadlines give your goals urgency.

Celebrate every success! Begin NOW.

CHAPTER 9
Step 5: Garbage in, Garbage out

Day 5:

Remember these:

- "I am in control of healing my concussion." (SILYMI)

- Keep eating Food that is your Medicine.

- "My Health is my NUMBER ONE priority." (SILYMI)

- Are you done creating your goals? If not, finish them.

- If yes, look at your goals first thing every morning.

All day long! Keep working – you're going to make it happen!

When you've completed this step, use the rate form from Chapter 4 to rate how you feel.

Congratulations! You're mid-way through the program! Thank your self for hanging in there!

You should be feeling progressively stronger. The first few steps built a foundation for you. You will NOW begin to make real changes in your life.

When it comes to your brain and to your normal outlook at life, do you feel more optimistic or more pessimistic? There's a lot of scientific evidence about how optimism and pessimism - expecting a positive or negative future - affects your brain. A growing pessimistic view makes you focus on what is bad in the world. So your brain focuses on that too.

What you focus on, grows. It's not hard to prove this. You just have to look at what and who you attract into your life. Like attracts like, just like a magnet! You just have to look at the things or circumstances that you have, that you like and don't like.

You must protect your optimistic outlook. In fact, if you don't think of yourself as particularly optimistic, you better start cultivating it now. Pessimism really does take a toll on your body. It takes a toll on your brain. It can make you notice negativity more often and put you, your body and therefore your brain, into stress mode.

In order to cut off the Sympathetic Nervous System, you need to take control of your emotional state. There are internal and external reasons to feel unhappy and stressed out. In this chapter, we'll deal with the things that happen or come from outside of you.

These things include negative newscasts, on the TV or radio or on the internet. They include the gossip you hear from your friends, either socially or at work. They may come from your family. This negativity may also come from people discouraging you from something you want or they make fun of you for wanting what you want!

I've certainly stopped watching the news and I am very choosy about the newspaper articles I read. I really only tune in to articles that might influence my business or my wellbeing. I'm curious about any new health developments to see how they compare to my work.

I've given up TV shows that are inherently negative, that philosophically contradict my beliefs about life. Or I remind myself that it's ONLY entertainment and don't get emotionally involved.

I've let go of friends who loved immersing themselves in drama or who are high maintenance. I will admit that in my earlier years, I was like that too. I've learned a lot from those experiences because I lost friendships that I valued.

Examine how you feel when you're around people. Which ones make you feel good? Which ones make you feel bad?

Consider this about dealing with the second group: *It's time to put those people aside, at least for the time being.* Or you may want to permanently leave them behind. Examine how you feel and be honest about it. It may be time to let these negative people out of your life.

You have to decide if your goals and your health are more important than pleasing these people. Remember your Number One priority. Your health includes your physical, mental and emotional health. If you don't feel upbeat with these people, then they're a drain to your energy and your sense of wellbeing.

Make a list of the things and people that have a negative impact on you, in whatever way that is. Then decide WHAT you will do about them. Then do it. Give yourself a deadline. *A deadline adds urgency.*

How do you know you're making the right decisions? When you make the right decisions, you feel good: You feel relieved and or happy. Your emotional state tells you everything you need to know.

When something isn't working out for you, look for the good in the situations that upset you or just plow through it and get it over with. Get the most distasteful things out of the way as soon as possible and be done with it! Do it NOW.

CHAPTER 10
Step 6: Create a Guarantee

Day 6:

Remember these:

- "I am in control of healing my concussion." (SILYMI)

- Keep eating Food that is your Medicine.

- "My Health is my NUMBER ONE priority." (SILYMI)

- Look at your goals first thing this morning.

- "I will only look for the positive aspects in my life." (SILYMI)

- Keep working on your goals

All day long! Keep up the good work!

When you've completed this step, use the rate form from Chapter 4 to rate how you feel.

I want you to create a mantra for yourself. Pick one of your goals and you will rephrase it in a short, positive, present-tense way.

For instance, several years ago, I learned that I can CONTROL my enjoyment on any trip that I take. The only reason to go on a trip is to ENJOY it, right? Why not GUARANTEE success? You really do have that much control!

So I say to myself, "I will arrive safely, on time, at my destination with my luggage intact at the same time."

Or if traveling with others: "We will arrive safely, on time, at our destination with our luggage intact at the same time."

It took a few rounds, even a few days, to get it right. My mantra, or other people call it an affirmation, had to contain all the elements to ensure a safe happy trip. When I said it, it had to feel right. It had to feel positive. I had to feel good when I said it. I also had to believe it. This all adds up to success.

When I finally got it the way I wanted it, I repeated it many, many times every day for weeks, if not months before the first trip I used it. Now because it's been many years, I repeat it to myself a few days or even just before leaving for the airport! When it is programmed into your brain, it doesn't take much activation any more, as long as you use it again.

It's your turn. Take one of your goals and do this:

- Word it in the present tense.

- Play with the words until it's short and easy to remember.

- Play with the words until it feels good to you and makes you feel confident.

- Write down the final version.

You may find that it still needs work. Do that until you've arrived at the right statements.

That's it. You can do that for each of your goals now. Start telling yourself these newly worded goals. Maybe some of your goals already sound right. Keep them the way they are. Again, this makes your brain focus on what's important to you. Begin NOW.

CHAPTER 11
Step 7: Time to Let Go of Certain Habits (of Thought)

Day 7 and beyond:

1. "I am in control of healing my concussion." (SILYMI)

2. Keep eating Food that is your Medicine.

3. "My Health is my NUMBER ONE priority." (SILYMI)

4. "I will only look for the positive aspects in my life." (SILYMI)

5. Declare your goals. (SILYMI)

6. Keep working on your goals

All day long! Good for you; keep it going!

When you've completed this step, use the rate form from Chapter 4 to rate how you feel.

Control is the power to restrain something, especially your own emotions or actions. Responsibility is an opportunity or ability to act independently and make decisions without authorization from someone else. This is autonomy!

Control and responsibility go hand in hand because what you can control and what you're responsible for are similar. Making this clear can help you release stress very quickly.

Here's what you can control. You have control over your thoughts, your feelings and emotions, your decisions, your actions and your results. These are the things you really have control over.

What are you responsible for? You're responsible for no one but yourself. So you're responsible for what you think, your feelings and emotions, the decisions you make, the actions you take and the results you get. Do you see how similar responsibility and control are?

The ONLY exception is when you have children that you are caring for. You are responsible to them and for them, until the age of majority, whatever that may be in your given jurisdiction. You have some control over them while they're young, but not total control.

Do you see, by exclusion, what you can't control or be responsible for?

You don't have control over other people, things, animals, situations or events. So, if you can't control everything that happens in your life, except yourself, then what is personal responsibility? You're not responsible for how someone else feels, thinks or does. For example, you're not responsible for making someone happy and they're not responsible for making you happy. You're responsible for your own happiness or unhappiness. It's the same for everyone else.

On the way back to Calgary after a wonderful week in Jamaica, we ran into a snag. We were very close to landing our flight when the pilot apologetically informed us that there was a major power outage at the Calgary International Airport. We were diverted to the Edmonton International Airport instead - a 20-minute plane ride north.

As usual there was the gamut of reactions. One man was sarcastic and upset. He was vocal. Other people silently stewed, with furrowed brows. The airline did the best they could.

That night I didn't react to the news of being diverted to Edmonton. I chose to be grateful that we had somewhere to land safely close by. On top of that, the plane had to refuel. It would've been bad if we were hundreds of miles away from an airport.

In Edmonton, the fueling truck came along and the driver tried to hook up the nozzle to the plane. Only to find out it was broken! As the pilot sheepishly announced another delay, people began to laugh. One guy piped up, "No problem, Mon!" and everyone laughed. People remembered their happy laid-back vacation in Jamaica.

We finally flew to Calgary and went to the carousel to pick up our luggage. We discovered that one piece was damaged. My husband immediately knew what to do. We headed straight to the Westjet customer service desk. They happily gave us a service order for repair or replacement. Then we finally headed home.

I realized what a LONG way I'd come. In years past, I would've been really upset, complaining loudly or sitting and stewing silently. Either way, it wouldn't have been good for me and certainly I wouldn't have made things easy on the flight crew (or my family) who were just doing their best keeping us abreast of the news. I wasn't going to let these little things make me forget the fun vacation I just had.

To help you in situations when you're negatively affected, find something about it that you can appreciate. I decided to appreciate having a refueling station so close. I appreciated the flight crew on that Westjet flight. I was grateful for a safe landing. I was grateful for the great holiday I just had.

This situation illustrates how to nip stress in the bud. There wasn't anything I could do, so helping myself remain calm was the best thing that I could do for me.

Even when there is more than one person involved, take full responsibility for your part in it. A really good example is road rage. When someone cuts you off in traffic, you might react. You might get angry. You might want to follow them home. But you know what? They didn't make you angry. You chose to be angry. And now, you're stressed out!

Surprises and requests for your patience and cooperation will still happen. That won't change. You're going to occasionally fall off the wagon. Just pick yourself up and dust yourself off. Don't make yourself feel worse by blaming yourself. You can say, "I have no control over this situation (this person, etc)."

Remind yourself that you are responsible for your results. (And for children if you have any.) Do so every hour for 5 minutes or in a cluster when you remember.

Celebrate each milestone. You can do it!

CHAPTER 12
Step 8: Resistance Is Futile

Day 8 and beyond:

1. "I am in control of healing my concussion." (SILYMI)

2. Keep eating Food that is your Medicine.

3. "My Health is my NUMBER ONE priority." (SILYMI)

4. "I will only look for the positive aspects in my life." (SILYMI)

5. Declare your goals. (SILYMI)

6. Keep working on your goals

7. Are you done with Step 7? If not, finish that before proceeding!

8. If yes, "I am responsible for the results I want." (SILYMI)

Keep it up – do the work; you're almost there...

When you've completed this step, use the rate form from Chapter 4 to rate how you feel.

Change can be a new or refreshingly different experience. You have to look at change differently. I truly hope that the reason why you're reading this book is that you're sincerely looking for solutions. And that means change.

Change is inevitable. This is a universal truth. As the Borg, in Star Trek, say, "Resistance is futile." Resistance creates stress. Change is always about growth even when it looks scary or negative. If you look at it this way, then you become adaptable and less stressed out.

For things to get better, you have to change. If you hope that other things outside of you change, then you'll be waiting a long time! Remember, you have no control over those external things.

If you want circumstances to change, then you've got to do it yourself.

Be adaptable. Be flexible. Be resilient. Being stubborn makes your miserable. You suffer when you refuse to adapt.

The body always follows the mind. Everyone is born with a weakness in certain parts of the body. So if they do everything right, with their thinking and feeling, with diet, exercise and rest, then everything falls into place. But if you do some things wrong, like having low self-esteem which leads to feeling helpless, then your weaker physical parts will be affected. In my son's case and yours, it was his head. Hence the concussion.

Change is going to happen regardless how you feel about it. Change is going to happen anytime, like in the airplane story in the last chapter. Anything can happen. If you can stop and make a decision to just go with the flow instead of resisting it, cursing it or trying to ignore it, you'll be much better off. And you'll know it, simply by how you feel.

When you come across something that you don't like, remind yourself that "Change is a new experience." Otherwise, do this every hour for 5 minutes or in a cluster when you remember. Celebrate each victory and know how far you've come along!

CHAPTER 13
Step 9: Needless Torture

Day 9 and beyond:

1. "I am in control of healing my concussion." (SILYMI)

2. Keep eating Food that is your Medicine.

3. "My Health is my NUMBER ONE priority." (SILYMI)

4. "I will only look for the positive aspects in my life." (SILYMI)

5. Declare your goals. (SILYMI)

6. Keep working on your goals

7. "I am responsible for the results I want." (SILYMI)

8. "Change is a new experience for me." (SILYMI)

All day long! Yes, great work!

When you've completed this step, use the rate form from Chapter 4 to rate how you feel.

A worry is a problem, cause for concern, issue, nuisance, pest, trouble, pain in the neck, headache, hassle and stress. Notice that a concussion often has bad headaches. There's a deeper meaning here. What are your headaches in life all about?

One of my son's worries was his new boss. The company had hired a new manager. At the very first team meeting this person told his group of young engineers that he wanted to be their friend!

That didn't go over well at all. In fact, one of his best friends at work declared – "I'm looking for another job!" He did find something and planned to move on. Nolan's reaction was just as quick, but it wasn't about quitting. In fact, it was the very opposite. He wanted to stay because there was an overwhelming number of reasons for him to stay. He enjoyed the way the company was managed. He enjoyed the actual work. He liked the people and the work environment. Leaving was not an option.

BUT he hated working for this guy!

So he was in a quandary. He couldn't make up his mind. He was confused.

A few months later, that's when the concussion happened. Nothing is actually an accident. Nothing ever happens randomly. There are always good reasons, mostly hidden to other people, but we FEEL it. That's ok. What's not ok is ignoring it and hoping it goes away. While we were working on my son's head injury, it became clear that the situation at work was a major issue for him.

So we worked on it together. Me gathering up the hard earned lessons I'd learned while in the corporate world and teaching them to my son. We came up with a plan and he had to execute it. It tested his resolve but he had to do what was necessary. Because he applied himself with new found courage and decisiveness, his effort led to the successful healing of his concussion.

Worry and anxiety activate your Sympathetic Nervous System. It sends out adrenaline and cortisol into your body and floods your brain. You can freeze if that's the right move or you can run. You're constantly in danger mode. That's exhausting to your nervous system.

WORRY ONLY MAKES THINGS WORSE! This is a personal

form of torture.

Worry and anxiety are about self-doubt and lack of self-confidence. You don't feel safe. Self-confidence comes from feeling safe. That's why you take risks. When you feel safe, you trust yourself.

Ambitious successful people learn how to deal with worry. So, I'm going to share a very good way to deal with worry in this chapter. My one-on-one students love this exercise.

It's time to pay attention to what's really on your mind. Whatever they are, they're probably not too far from the surface. Deal with them now. Grab a piece of paper.

Write WORRIES at the top of the page. Use the following categories to help you look at each area of your life:

- Physical (mobility, injuries, pain, digestive, appetite, breathing, etc.)

- Emotional (sleep, how much, depression, etc.)

- Spiritual

- Relationships (family, extended family, in-laws, marriage, parenthood, children, lovers, friends, enemies, co-workers, bosses, subordinates, business partners, vendors, clients, teachers, instructors, etc.)

- Career or job

- Recreation

- Business, if you have one as an entrepreneur or you're deeply involved in the operations of a business.

- School, if you're a student.

- Pets

- Situations

- Events

Deal with your worry and concerns. Don't let them fester.

For each worry or concern, do this:

- State whether you have control over this or not.

- State whether you have responsibility for it or not.

Eliminate the items where you have no direct control or responsibility.

Prioritize what you have left, starting with the most important.

State what evidence you have for each item in your original list. That's right, what evidence do you have that something bad is going to happen? You may be surprised. It certainly surprises my one-on-one students! They are often stumped because they suddenly can't think of a reason why they're worried! Then the feeling goes away.

Now, what's left? Write down why you want it changed. A compelling reason makes desire for change very strong. If there is none, then maybe it's really not important.

If it is important, then quickly write down a plan. Set a deadline. Deadlines add urgency! This exercise is a reality check. You're taking control. It deflates a lot of stress. You take control only if you take action. So do something NOW about your worries.

The result of getting rid of stress is you begin to feel the opposite:

Confident.

Safe.

Self-sufficient.

Brave.

Courageous, in fact.

Decisive.

Much, much better!

Celebrate each victory! How does your self-rating look now?

CHAPTER 14
Step 10: What Drives Your Crazy?

Day 10 and beyond:

1. "I am in control of healing my concussion." (SILYMI)

2. Keep eating Food that is your Medicine.

3. "My Health is my NUMBER ONE priority." (SILYMI)

4. "I will only look for the positive aspects in my life." (SILYMI)

5. Declare your goals. (SILYMI)

6. Keep working on your goals

7. "I am responsible for the results I want." (SILYMI)

8. " Change is a new experience for me." (SILYMI)

9. Keep working on each item in your worries list. FEEL good about it!

10. You're on the home stretch!

When you've completed this step, use the rate form from Chapter 4 to rate how you feel..

When I talk about tolerations with my clients for the first time, they look at me with a blank face. They never considered this before. What are they and why should you be concerned about them?

Tolerations are the things that bug you. Some of them are minor irritations. Some create major upset. Some may only bug you once in a while when you come across it and then you remember. Or there are daily reminders about others. But they bug you.

Tolerations rob you of time, space, energy and resources. If you're tolerating anything, it takes away your harmony and peace of mind. Complaining and blaming about them only reinforces a negative emotional state and mindset.

Anything can bug you: things, people, events, situations, the job, the career or animals that we put up with everyday of your life. Maybe you've been told to suck it up, baby. It's part of the job. That's life, etc.

You don't have to tolerate anything that you don't like in your life. You can change anything to your liking, however you must take full responsibility to make the changes. Expecting others to do it for you when you're not willing to change it yourself only makes you feel worse. And you'll be waiting for a long time. And you'll have to ACCEPT the solution that someone else has created. So take control of them yourself! You're trying to reduce stress, remember?

Here's your reward: Whenever you eliminate something from your life, you make room for something much better. You'll feel lighter.

List as many tolerations as you can. Here are some clues to help you gather your thoughts:

What do you spend time complaining about? What do you spend time blaming others for?

Tolerations may also be the hot buttons that set you off. Perhaps some of your tolerations are also on the worry list. Or they're already one of your goals that you set earlier.

Prioritize your top 10. Transfer those to a blank sheet of paper or organize them in your spreadsheet.

Ask yourself again if you have control over these things. Ask yourself if you're responsible for them. If you answer No to BOTH these questions, then strike them off the list immediately!

With what's left, what positive action or actions will you take to address each item in that priority list? When it comes to taking positive action, you can do a number of things with them. It doesn't matter if it's a thing, animal, a relationship, a job, a career, etc.

You're choosing to have peace and harmony:

- Eliminate it.

- End it.

- Transform it.

- Change it.

- Give it away.

- Donate it.

- Use it a different way.

- Leave it.

- Create a new perspective, look at it a different way.

- Decide to do your best.

- Take charge.

- Take control.

- Move away.

- Etc.

If you thought of other creative things to do with your list, include those ideas. Being creative and feeling in control are good things. Some of the things on your list are going to require courage, like leaving a job or career that no longer engages you. It may not look like a positive thing at first, but any feelings of stress indicates that you're NOT happy about it anyways.

Give yourself a deadline for each item; otherwise NOTHING is going to change. These exercises will empower you. Then you're no longer a victim, but becoming a victor.

Finish the work. Get it done. Keep working on each of your worries and on each of your tolerations. It may take a while to get through the list, but strike each one off as you come to a RESOLUTION for each one. The more you strike off, the more LIGHTER you will feel. The fewer HEADACHES you will literally have. The more clarity you will feel because your mind is no longer cluttered by all this junk.

Celebrate each toleration that you cross off your list!

Prologue

More than 4 years ago, when we heard that the 2014 World Cup of Soccer would be held in Brazil, Nolan & I said, "We're going!" Brazil is our favorite international soccer team. It was a no-brainer. My husband and my youngest son, not so much. But we planned a family trip for four anyways. I said we're going to Brazil and we're going to have a great time whether we get tickets are not.

We knew we wanted to see games after the 32-team group stage. We picked out one location instead of traveling. We knew the weather there was going to be hot and humid. So we wanted to be near a beach in between games. We had our criteria and wrote it all down. We knew what we wanted. We had well defined goals. And then we quashed every doubt, ignored every piece of bad news about the tournament. (Did you spot any of my declarations in these two paragraphs?)

We applied for the ticket lottery in August 2013. At this time, FIFA hadn't picked out the teams in each group yet so we didn't know which teams we were going to see. We looked for accommodations and flights and booked and paid for it all up front in October 2013 and then we waited for the lottery results in November. Then we invited some over-seas friends who were also crazy Brazil fans to meet us.

When the time FINALLY arrived, we were ALL excited! It was the BEST vacation that I ever had. It worked out perfectly.

Nolan, being perfectly healthy and by then, about 19 months concussion free, was able to make choices. He did exactly what he wanted – he was the guy who won the ticket lottery for our family! It was a complete thrill to be part of this major international sporting event.

You too, can have your life back and have all the choices you want to live a full life.

Change yourself and you change your circumstances.

The lesson here is that whenever something you don't like happens, you want something different. You want it the way it will make you happy. So, you have to make the changes - in yourself. You have the right and the ability to make positive changes in your life. If you try to change something external to yourself, you're going to be very unhappy and stressed out for a very long time. Mentally. Emotionally. Physically.

I know that Nolan wasn't always willing to follow everything I instructed him to do, because it was outside of his comfort zone. But I wouldn't let him off the hook. Take positive action where you can. Sometimes it's scary. Sometimes it's going to take a lot of courage. Sometimes it'll be a No-Brainer! But you'll know if it's the right thing for you to do.

You can be well again. I know you're already well on your way, if you applied this program. You cannot fail when you're focused and have the drive to succeed! I wish you all the best! Thanks for being courageous.

CELEBRATE!

The Ten Steps ends here, but your work may continue. It depends on how willing and consistent you were, following the program. Your past doesn't matter. But how you conduct yourself each day that you work on the program does.

Perhaps some of the work that you uncover will take longer than 21 days to resolve. That's ok. But do NOT stop working at those things. It's so critical to your wellbeing.

Continue to work on the items that matter to you. Maybe you'll even realize that they weren't as important to you as you thought. In any case, don't think about what you've lost as a result of your concussion. Think about your goals instead. Do not permit a re-entry into your past life, because that's not who you are now.

No, what you're aiming for now is to grow stronger. You must, because you were weak for some reason when the concussion happened. If you've followed the Ten Steps you are far stronger now than you were then.

If you haven't recovered fully yet, repeat the program, this time with even more determination. It just means you need some more time. That's ok too.

I have one small request of you. If you found that this book has helped you in any way, please go to Amazon and write a nice simple review about what it did for you. You see, if it helped you at all, then this message must go out to others who also need the same help. There must be thousands out there, some desperate for answers. Please pay it forward with a simple review. You could be helping many others achieve their goal for wellness after a concussion. Thank you so much!

CELEBRATE! All the best in your endeavors. I know you can be well again!

For Further Reading

1. Dispenza, Joe, DC, *Evolve Your Brain* (Deerfield, Florida: Health Communications, Inc., 2007)

2. Rankin, Lissa MD, *Mind Over Medicine* (Carlsbad, California: Hay House, 2013), pp. 233–252.

3. Lu, Henry C., PhD, *Chinese System of Food Cures* (Sterling Publishing Co., Inc: New York)

4. Pitchford, Paul, L.Ac, *Healing with Whole Foods, Third Edition* (Berkeley, California: North Atlantic Books, 2002, Third Revision)

5. Liu, Joanny Dr., *Knock OUT Concussions* (Vervante, 2013)

6. Liu, Joanny Dr., *Rapid Injury Recovery: How Elite Athletes Use Sports Psychology to Heal FAST and Have a Long Stable Career* (Harmoni Health Inc, 2015)

CPSIA information can be obtained
at www.ICGtesting.com
Printed in the USA
LVHW021646110619
620865LV00016B/1246

9 780994 015020